Beyonce Recipes Book 2:

17 Delicious Recipes For Weight Loss and Healthy Living

By

Brittany Samons

Table of Contents

Introduction 5
1. Spanish Tortilla Recipe 7
2. Zucchini with Tomatoes Recipe 8
3. Shepherd's Pie Recipe 10
4. Vegetables and Lentil Soup Recipe 12
5. Chickpea Mock Tuna Salad Recipe 14
6. Venison Stew Recipe 16
7. Pinto Bean Soup Recipe 18
8. Sautéed Zucchini Recipe 21
9. Butternut Squash Puree with Pecans Recipe .. 22
10. Roasted Egg Plant Dip Recipe 24
11. Black Bean Dip Recipe 26
12. Pumpkin Soup Recipe 28
13. Pumpkin Cake Recipe 30
14. Mini Vegetables Frittatas Recipe 32
15. Turkey Burger Recipe 34
16. Steamed Chicken and Vegetables 36
17. Seasoned Wilted Spinach Recipe 38
Final Words 39
Thank You Page 40

Beyond Diet Recipes Book 2:

17 Delicious Recipes For Weight Loss and Healthy Living

By Brittany Samons

© Copyright 2014 Brittany Samons

Reproduction or translation of any part of this work beyond that permitted by section 107 or 108 of the 1976 United States Copyright Act without permission of the copyright owner is unlawful. Requests for permission or further information should be addressed to the author.

This publication is designed to provide accurate and authoritative information in regard to the subject matter covered. This work is sold with the understanding that the publisher is not engaged in rendering legal, accounting, or other professional services. If legal advice or other expert assistance is required, the services of a competent professional person should be sought.

First Published, 2014

Printed in the United States of America

Introduction

The importance of health can be perceived by this saying that "Health is wealth", but this saying has become more important and realized in a couple of decades. The threat of different diseases have increased, some of which are quite life threatening like cardiac diseases. This increase risk has also make people more conscious of their health and they have started to strive for the change to make their health better or even revive it for some extent.

Well once health is gone, it's hard to restore it in its natural form. Now you may be thinking then what is the solution? If you are facing the issue of overweight and looking for to get in best health. The best thing suggested by the doctors and health consultant is to take care of your body by looking over the things to give it or feed it to provide it with all the luxurious comfort. Be careful, maybe you are feeding your body with wrong things which may seem right to you.

Yes, it is possible that you are not really doing the right thing to keep yourself in good health. Feeding your body with fast food and over eating is the simplest example. Not each everything you eat is really good for you. If you do not pay attention to what is right for you, then you will definitely push your health into the threatening zone. Having a slim body to show off on hot summer at beach and to fit in the smallest size must not be good to have your only goal. Your first priority must be to have a healthy body. When you have a healthy body, your body will remain in shape automatically.

1. Spanish Tortilla Recipe

Ingredients:

-1 diced Onion (large)

- 5 Eggs

- 1 pound of Potatoes

- ¼ cup of olive oil

- Salt and Pepper according to taste

Directions to prepare:

Take the potatoes and cut them into thin slices. Take a pan and put it over medium flame, add in it the olive oil, onion and potatoes. Sauté them until golden brown. It will take approximately 3 minutes.

Take the eggs in the bowl, add in it the salt and pepper. Beat the eggs with the hand or electronic beater until foamy. Now pour the eggs over the potatoes and onions in the pan. Cover the pan and let it cook on low heat for 6 – 7 minutes. If the bottom is golden brown and omelet is set. Flip it with the wooden spatula or spoon to cook the upper layer for 4 – 5 minutes. Once cooked well now take it off in the plate, cut it and serve as desire. The delicious Spanish tortilla is ready to make your breakfast the healthier and yummiest.

2. Zucchini with Tomatoes Recipe

Ingredients:

-3/4 teaspoon of salt

- 2 tablespoon of olive oil

- 2 peeled, and copped medium tomatoes

- ½ teaspoon of black pepper (grounded)

- 2 washed and trimmed medium size zucchini

- 2 tablespoon of butter

- 1 or 2 minced garlic cloves

- 2 chopped medium size onions

½ teaspoon of dried thyme

Direction for Preparation:

Take the zucchini wash and dry it. Cut it lengthwise into quarters. Then further slice each quarter into rounds quarters. Mix it with the salt and set aside for an hour. Now rinse the zucchini and left for some time to dry properly.

Take a pan or skillet and add in it the 1 table spoon of butter and olive oil each. Put the pan over medium flame. Add the zucchini in the pan and sauté it until golden. Take off the zucchini from the pan into a bowl or plate. Now add the onions and 1 table spoon of olive oil and butter each in the pan. Again place the pan over the medium flame and let the onion cook for some minutes until tender. Now add the tomatoes in it and cook it for some time until all the water get absorbed. Add the thyme, garlic, pepper and cooked zucchini in the onion and tomatoes mixture. Mix all the ingredients well and sauté it for 1 minute to ensure everything get mix well. Be careful, do not overcook the zucchini. Enjoy the zucchini with some different flavor.

3. Shepherd's Pie Recipe

Ingredients:

- 2 minced garlic cloves
- 1 chopped tomato (large)
- 3 cups of legumes (cooked)
- 1 teaspoon of soy sauce pepper (gluten free)
- 2 ½ tablespoon of olive oil
- 3 cups of finely chopped mixed vegetables
- ½ cup of chopped onion
- 2 – 21/2 cup of mashed cauliflower
- 1 cup of vegetable water or stock

Instructions:

Take a pan and put it over medium heat, add in it the 2 tablespoon of olive oil and minced garlic, sauté them for about 2 minutes. Now add the chopped onion in it and sauté again until the onion get soft. It may take 5 more minutes. Once the onion are done add in it the tomatoes and cook for 2 minutes, stir frequently and if you like then you can mashed the tomatoes too. Then add the vegetable stock, cover the pan and let it boil until all the vegetables get cooked completely or tender to touch. The vegetables may take 5 – 10 minutes to cook properly.

Now add in it the soy sauce, salt and pepper to taste. Now heat the oven at 350 F. Take a pie plate and grease it with ½ tablespoon of olive oil. Pour in the vegetables and top with the layer of the mashed potatoes. Garnish it and bake for 30 minutes. Serve the shepherd's pie hot and enjoy the new veggie taste.

4. Vegetables and Lentil Soup Recipe

Ingredients:

- 1 cup of chopped onion
- 2 cups of shredded cabbage
- 3 chopped carrots
- 1 teaspoon of salt
- ½ teaspoon of basil (dried)
- ¼ teaspoon of curry powder
- ½ cup of green and red lentils
- 2 cups of chicken broth
- ½ teaspoon of grounded black pepper
- 1 stalk chopped celery
- 1 can of tomatoes chopped
- 1 cup of chopped onions
- 1 crushed garlic clove
- ½ teaspoon of thyme dried

Instruction for Preparation:

Take a large bowl, add in it the lentils and twice the depths of the lentils add in it the water. Now place the bowl in the oven and boil it for 15 minutes or until the lentils get cooked. Now drain the extra water from the lentils and rinse them. Add in it the celery, chicken broth, onion, tomatoes, carrots, cabbage and garlic. Season it with the thyme, pepper, salt, curry and basil. Cook for more 1 – 2 hours all the things get cooked properly. Serve the soap hot and enjoy this delicious soap on cold nights.

5. Chickpea Mock Tuna Salad Recipe

Ingredients:

- 1/2 cup of sunflower seeds
- Water as required
- 2 tablespoon of lemon juice
- 2 teaspoon of olive oil or flaxseed oil
- ½ cup of mayonnaise
- 1/3 cup of minced or chopped red onion
- ½ cup of almonds
- 1 cup of canned, cooked or soaked chickpeas
- ¼ cup of sesame seeds
- 1 tablespoon of soy sauce (gluten free)
- 1 – 2 teaspoon of kelp powder
- 2 tablespoon of freshly minced parsley
- 1 minced celery stalk

Instructions to Prepare:

First of all rinse the seeds and almonds properly, use a small holed sieve to carefully wash the seeds especially the sesame seeds. Now put them all in a bowl and pour water until seeds get soaked completely in the water. Cover the bowl and set it aside overnight so that the seeds get soaked properly. Then rinse and drain all the water.

Take food processor and add in it the almonds, lemon juice, soy sauce, olive oil, kelp powder, water, seeds and chickpeas. Blend all the ingredients will for 1 – 2 minutes until turn into a smooth paste.

Now take a bowl and add in it the celery, parsley, onion, and mayonnaise and chickpea mixture. Cover the bowl and place it in refrigerator or at least 30 minutes.

You can keep this tuna salad in the refrigerator for 2 – 3 days. Enjoy the tuna salad and stay healthy.

6. Venison Stew Recipe

Ingredients:

-1 pinch of salt
- 1 tablespoon of coconut oil
- 1 medium chopped red onion
- 2 teaspoon of dried thyme
- 1 teaspoon of orange zest
- 3 cups of beef stock
- 1 ½ pound of stewing venison
- 1 pinch of freshly ground black pepper
- 3 sliced stalk of celery
- 1 teaspoon of ground cinnamon
- 3 medium chopped and peeled kohlrabi
- ½ cup of fresh cranberries

Directions:

Take venison and season it with the salt and pepper. Take a pan, add in it the coconut oil and place it over the medium heat. Add in it the onion and sauté until the onion get tender, translucent and soft. Take off the vegetables and set aside.

Now add the venison in the pan and sauté until turn into golden brown. Then add in it the dried thyme, orange zest, stock, cinnamon, cranberries and kohlrabi and mix all of them well. Add in it the sautéed vegetables and cook again. Let the mixture heat until it starts to bubble or cook for 45 – 50 minutes. When all the vegetables and venison get tender, remove the pan from the heat and take off the venison stew in a plate and serve hot.

7. Pinto Bean Soup Recipe

Ingredients:

- 1 small butternut squash or a large yam
- Half head of cauliflower
- ½ teaspoon of dried ginger or 2 thin slices of fresh ginger
- 1 teaspoon of mustard seed (brown)
- 1 teaspoon of ground coriander seed
- 1 bay leaf
- ½ teaspoon of turmeric
- ½ teaspoon of fennel
- 2/3 cup of coconut milk
- 2 cups of water
- 1 tablespoon of soy sauce (gluten free)
- ½ teaspoon of fresh ground black pepper
- 2 tablespoon of olive oil
- 3 stalks of celery
- 1 pinch of cayenne or 1 seeded jalapeno pepper
- 1 – 2 raw garlic cloves
- ½ teaspoon of ground cumin seeds
- 1 teaspoon of paprika
- 2 teaspoon of dry or fresh basil leaves
- 2 cups of cooked pinto beans

- 1 teaspoon of ground coriander seeds
- ½ cinnamon stick
- Salt to taste or ½ teaspoon of salt
- ¼ cup of fresh chopped parsley leaves

Directions for Preparation:

Take a large pan, Pour in it the little bit of olive oil and add coconut milk, pinto beans, veggie cube, bay leaf, water and cinnamon stick. Sauté all the ingredients on low heat. Add the minced ginger, garlic and jalapeno pepper. Also add mustard seeds all the veggies except cauliflower in the oil. Cook them for 10 minutes.

Take the ½ cauliflower, remove the steam and leaves. Cut it into cubical pieces and set aside. Now add the cauliflower an all the other remaining spices in the pan and let them cook for few more minutes.

Now add the water, beans and coconut oil in the pan already containing all the things previously added. Cover the pan and let it cook on low heat. Once all the vegetables get tender to touch and soup get thickened, add in it the salt, pepper, freshly chopped parsley and soy sauce. Stir the soup well and let it cook for more couple of minutes.

Remove the pan from the heat and serve hot in the bowls. This soup is full of protein and nutrients and a great meal for cold winter nights and evening. It is also of low calories and will keep you full for longer.

8. Sautéed Zucchini Recipe

Ingredients:

- 2 teaspoon of sea salt
- 1/2 lemon juice
- 6 washed and trimmed medium zucchini
- 2 tablespoon of olive oil or butter
- Ground black pepper to taste
- Sea salt to taste

Instructions:

Take the zucchini and rinse them well. Cue the zucchini into the thin slices. Now put all the slices zucchini into a bowl and add in it the salt. Mix the salt well with the zucchini and set it aside for an hour. After an hour rinse the zucchini and pat dry.

Take a pan and put it on the low heat. Add in it the olive oil or butter and also the sliced zucchini. Sauté the zucchini in the pan for about one minute. Take a plate and place the sautéed zucchini in it. Seasoned with salt, pepper and lemon juice.

9. Butternut Squash Puree with Pecans Recipe

Ingredients:

- 3 slightly beaten eggs
- Sea salt, to taste
- 3 butternut squash, medium
- 2 table spoon of melted butter
- 1 -2 tablespoon of butter
- ¾ cup of chopped raw pecans
- ¼ teaspoon of nutmeg

Instructions for Preparation:

Take the squash and cut it into half and remove all the seeds. Preheat the oven at 350F. Take a baking dish and fill it with the ½ inch of water and place the squash in it. Place the baking dish into the oven and let it cook for an hour until squash get tender.

Now pour the squash into a blender and process in until turn into a smooth mixture. Now add in it the beaten eggs, salt and nutmeg. Now pour the puree into a baking dish. Add in it the melted butter and sprinkle the pecans over it. Place the baking dish into the oven and let it cook for more 30 minutes. After 30 minutes remove the baking dish from the oven and serve hot.

10. Roasted Egg Plant Dip Recipe

Ingredients:

-1 table spoon of Olive Oil

- ½ Cup of fresh lemon juice

- 2 Minced garlic cloves

- 2 lbs of eggplant

- 4 tablespoon of yogurt

- 4 tablespoon of tahini

Instructions to Follow:

Take the eggplant and cut into halves. Take each halve and further cut lengthwise to expose the face. Now brush the face of each piece with the olive oil. Preheat the oven at 450F and place the eggplant face up in the baking dish and cook until tender, soft and black.

If you are want to grill it then Place the eggplant face down on the cooking grill and cook it for 50 minutes on until get soft and black. Once cooked, place them on the platter to cool down.

Take a spoon and remove the flesh of the eggplant and put it into the food processor. Blend it on low speed until turn into a mixture. Now mix in it the lemon juice, salt, tahini and other ingredients and place it in refrigerator for an hour.

Take a bowl and pour the mixture in it and sprinkle over it the olive oil and parsley. You can serve it with the vegetables and whatever you like.

Tips: You can store it into a refrigerator for 2 – 3 days, but if you are planning to store it, then it's better to use less amount of garlic clove, as they get hard in the refrigerator. Grilling is the best way to adopt for cooking eggplant as it makes the eggplant more smoky and rich in taste.

11. Black Bean Dip Recipe

Ingredients:

- ½ cup of hot water
- 1 teaspoon of coriander (ground)
- ¼ cup of chopped cilantro
- 2 – 3 lemon (juice)
- 2 c canned, drained and soaked black beans
- 1 teaspoon of cumin (ground)
- 1 teaspoon of chipotle chile
- 1 tablespoon of olive oil
- 1 – ½ teaspoon of salt, or salt to taste
- ¼ cup of sliced scallions

Instructions to prepare:

Take a bowl and put in it the black beans and water until the water is quite higher than beans. Let them sit for some time. Now pour 1 tablespoon of olive oil in a pan and put it over medium flame. Add in it the cumin, coriander and scallions. Sauté it for 10 minutes or until tender.

Now add this mixture, Chile, spices and cilantro in the beans. Also add the lime juice and salt as per requirement. Keep this bean dip in the refrigerator for at least 5 days. Always serve hot as it taste better when hot or at room temperature.

12. Pumpkin Soup Recipe

Ingredients:

-1 washed, trimmed and cut into rings leek
- 1 qt of vegetable stock
- 1 teaspoon of pepper, or taste
- 1 ½ pounds pumpkin
- 2 tablespoon of olive oil
- 1 – ½ teaspoon of cayenne pepper
- 2 sliced and peeled potatoes
- ½ teaspoon of salt, or to taste

Instructions for Preparation:

Take the pumpkin and cut its top. Remove the seeds and strings from the inside. Peel off the hard shell and carefully sliced the flesh. Put the pan at medium heat, add in it the olive oil, potatoes, leek and pumpkin. Sauté them all by constant stirring for 5 minutes.

Now add in the vegetables stock and let it boil for some time. Potatoes will take more time to cook so cover the pan and let it boil until potatoes get soft. Once the potatoes and other ingredients get cooked well, add in it the remaining spices and lemon juice. Stir the soup well and serve hot in the bowl.

Tips: Use small and flavored pumpkins for better tasted soup. By carefully cutting the pumpkin you can use its leftover for lantern or making any other useful thing.

13. Pumpkin Cake Recipe

Ingredients:

- 3 tablespoon of coconut flour
- Orange zest to taste or 1 pinch
- 1 pinch of cardamom, or to taste
- ½ teaspoon of baking soda
- 6 – 8 eggs
- 1 pinch of cinnamon or to taste
- ¼ teaspoon of vanilla
- 1 can of organic pumpkin
- 1 pinch of fresh ginger (grated), or to taste

Directions to Follow:

Take all the ingredients and mix them well until a smooth foamy batter will form. Now put the pan over the medium low heat, add in it a little bit of coconut or olive oil. Now carefully pour the small amount of the mixture into the pan and cook until bubbles are started to form on the surface.

Now by using wooden spoon or spatula flip the pancake and cook the other surface. Once the pancake turn light brown take it off into a plate.

Now pour the remaining mixture into the pan and cook it following the same procedure as previously. Serve hot by using fruits syrup. Enjoy the delicious and healthy pumpkin pancakes.

14. Mini Vegetables Frittatas Recipe

Ingredients:

-1 tablespoon of butter

- 1 cup of diced red pepper

- 1 diced leek

- 1 teaspoon of sea salt

- 1 cup of diced zucchini

- ¼ cup of fresh parsley

- 8 large eggs

- 1 cup of sliced fresh mushrooms

- ½ teaspoon of black pepper

- ½ cup of raw organic milk

Instructions for Preparation:

Take a large muffin tin or mold, grease it with the butter. Take a bowl and whisk in it the eggs and milk till a foamy mixture is formed. Now set aside this mixture.

Preheat the oven at 350 F. Take a pan or skillet and place it in the medium heat, add in it the butter. Once the butter get melt, add in it the zucchini, mushrooms, leek and red pepper. Sauté these all until the vegetables get soft or sauté them for 5 minutes.

Now remove the pan from the heat and add in it the parsley. Stir the mixture well and also add in it the pepper and salt to taste. Add the vegetables in the egg mixture and mix well.

Now pour this mixture into the muffin tin or cups. Bake them in the oven for 20 – 30 minutes until the frittatas get brown on the top. You can serve them hot, but if you want to eat them later then store them in the refrigerator for later use.

15. Turkey Burger Recipe

Ingredients:

- 2 slices of tomato
- 3 leaves of lettuce
- 4 slices of cucumber
- 1/8 teaspoon of garlic powder
- 2 slices of bacon
- 5 oz. of ground lean turkey
- 1 swg bread
- Pepper to taste
- salt to taste
- Cheddar cheese (raw)
- 1 table spoon of coconut oil
- 1/2 sliced avocado

Directions to follow:

Take a nonstick pan and add in it 1 tablespoon of coconut oil. Put the pan over a medium heat. Take turkey garlic, salt and pepper and mix them all well. Make the round burger patties and cook them in the pan until it puff up and turn golden brown or cook them for 6 minutes at least. Add in it the cheese and bacon.

Now take the bread and place the avocado slices over it. Also top it with the turkey patties, tomatoes, slices of cucumber. Also place the lettuce leaves over it, now put another bread over it and enjoy the healthy turkey burger with any good fruit drink.

16. Steamed Chicken and Vegetables

Ingredients:

-1 ginger root cut and slices into think sticks.

- 6 green onions of scallions chopped.

- ¾ cup of lengthwise cut baby carrots

- 2 teaspoon of coconut oil

- 1 teaspoon of salt, or to taste

- 1 medium chopped garlic clove

- 2 large cut in halves boneless chicken breast

- ½ cup of chicken stock

- ½ cup of chopped parsley

- Ground black pepper to taste

Instructions for Preparation:

You can cook in the Bundt pan or bamboo streamer tray. Use as per your convenience.

Take a large stock pot and add in it the 2 -3 inches of water and let it boil. Once the water get boiled, lower the heat. Add the shredded cabbage at the bottom of the Bundt pan. Take a large bowl and add in it the chicken breasts, ginger, parsley, garlic, carrots and scallions. Mix them all together. Now add in it the salt, pepper and oil. Toss the mixture to mix all the spices too. Put the mixture over the cabbage carefully. Now place the Bundt pan into the water boiling in stock pot.

Place the chicken stock over the mixture of vegetables and chicken. Cover the Bundt pan and let it cook for 20 minutes. After 20 minutes uncover the pan and check with fork if chicken breast are get cooked or not. If it is done, take off the pan from the stock pot and serve the steamy chicken with vegetables hot. Enjoy the healthy chicken roasted without oil.

17. Seasoned Wilted Spinach Recipe

Ingredients:

-1 tablespoon of butter

- 1 tablespoon of pine nuts

- 2 bunches of fresh spinach

- 1 minced garlic clove

- 1 tablespoon of dried tomato flakes

Instructions for Preparation:

Take spinach and wash it under tap water carefully. Now cut and remove the stem of the spinach. Take a large pot and put spinach in it. Place the pot or pan over medium heat. Cover and cook the spinach until it get wilted. Do not add water into the spinach while cooking as the water spinach already contained will be enough to cook it.

Take a pan and melt in it the butter and add tomatoes flakes, garlic and nuts in it. Now pour it over the spinach and mix them well. Serve them in a plate and enjoy the healthy veggie food.

Final Words

If you are a diet conscious person, then it's not a bad thing to hide as it is good to be careful towards your health. You all energy, activities and even success depends upon your health. By eating the right diet and in balanced amount, is the things through which you can reward yourself a productive and healthy life, which is not only beneficial for yourself but for others too.

These above mentioned recipes are specially designed, to help you provide your body with the right amount and kind of nutrients. The use of vegetables and fruits especially in raw form are quite important to guarantee the efficient function of your body organs. It will also protect you from many life threatening diseases like cardiac attacks etc. Vegetables are fat free and full of healthy nutrients.

Thank You Page

I want to personally thank you for reading my book. I hope you found information in this book useful and I would be very grateful if you could leave your honest review about this book. I certainly want to thank you in advance for doing this.

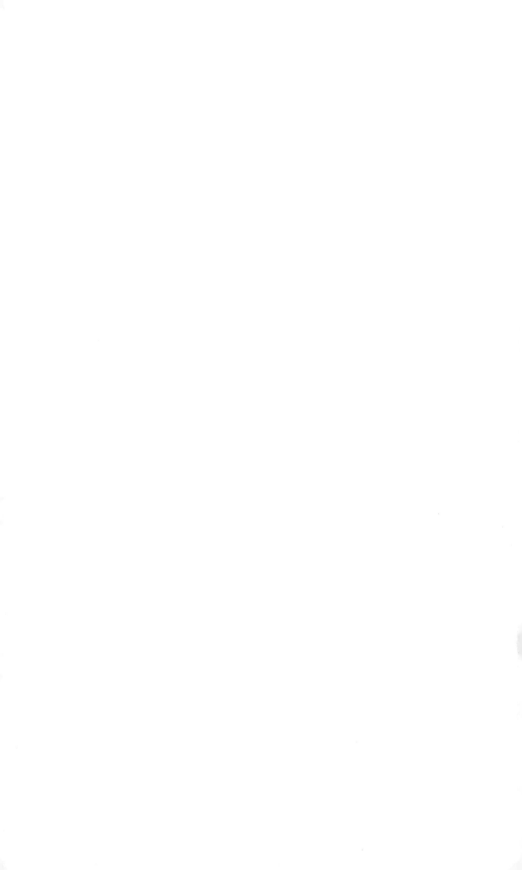

Lightning Source UK Ltd.
Milton Keynes UK
UKOW06f1949210715

255601UK00013B/403/P